The Year My Dad Went Bald

A tale of cancer, chemo
and coping with a cold head

*Written & illustrated
by Brian Kraft*

To Brigid
Best Wishes!
Brian Kraft

The Year My Dad Went Bald

Text and illustration copyright © 2010 by Brian Kraft
All right reserved. No part of this book may be reproduced or transmitted in any form or by any means, electronic or mechanical, without the express written consent from the author or his authorized agent, except in the case of brief excerpts in critical reviews and articles. All inquiries should be addressed to:

Brian Kraft
46 Webster Park Ave.
Columbus, OH 43214
kraft.42@osu.edu

Printed by Bang Printing, Brainerd, Minn., United State of America

Library of Congress Cataloging-in-Publication Data
Kraft, Brian (1966)
    The Year My Dad Went Bald / by Brian Kraft – 1st edition
    [36] p
Summary: A hockey-playing boy and his family cope with his father's cancer diagnosis, treatment and recovery.
ISBN: 978-0-615-42154-4
1. Cancer—juvenile literature. 2. Lymphoma. 3. Youth hockey

We acknowledge with the utmost thanks and appreciation the work of those who supported us through the challenges of our cancer diagnosis and treatment, including the Columbus Blue Jackets and its charitable Foundation, the Leukemia and Lymphoma Society, Ohio Health's Cancer Care, Dr. Andrew Grainger of Columbus Oncology and Hematology Associates, Dr. Jennifer Ball of the Columbus Clinic of Naturopathy, Dr. Mark Varckette of Varckette Family Chiropractic, Mary Anne Linder of Linder Acupuncture, our Columbus Ice Hockey Club family, and the NHL and National Hockey League Players' Association's Hockey Fights Cancer effort.

A portion of all profits from the sale of this book will be donated to Hockey Fights Cancer, and the Leukemia and Lymphoma Society.

CPSIA facility code: BP 305786

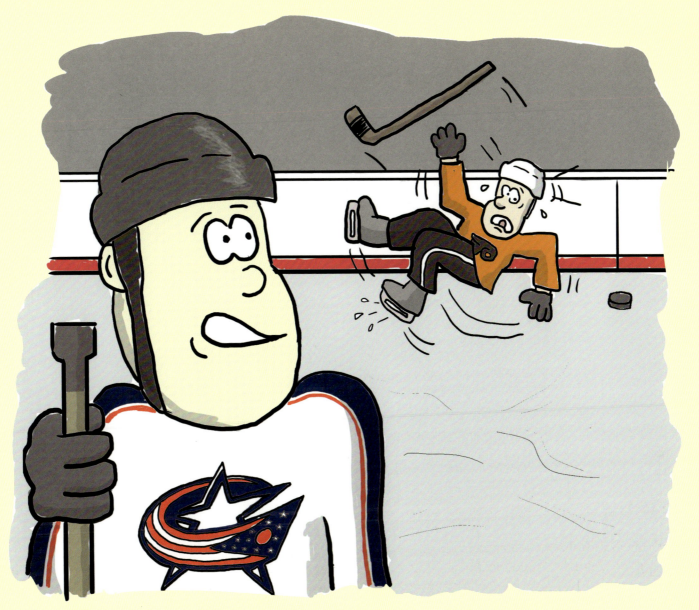

That's my Dad over there. He's not the best hockey player or even that good of a skater. But it is great to see him on the ice. For a while, I wasn't sure I would ever see him out here again. A couple of months ago he wasn't feeling so good and went to see his doctor. His back was hurting badly, and he thought he had injured it somehow. The news he got was much worse.

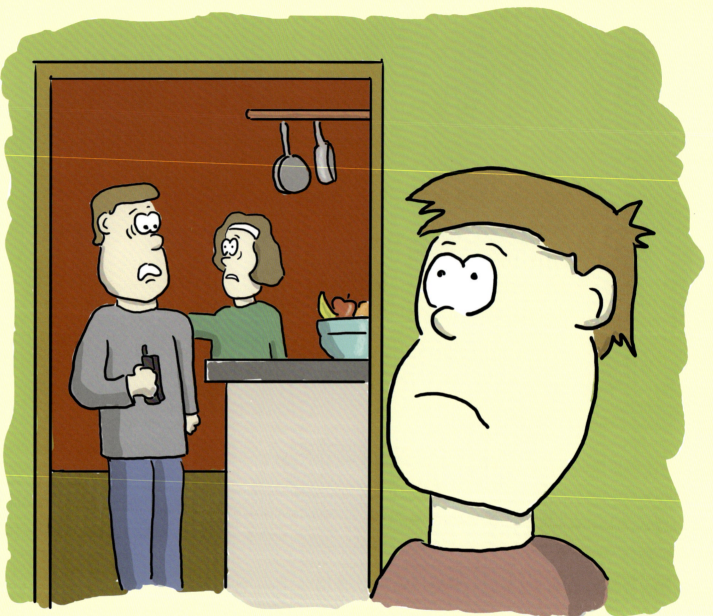

After school one day, Dad got a call from his doctor, and I could tell that the news wasn't good.

He and mom were talking in the kitchen, and they sounded worried.

I was getting nervous when they came out to tell me what was going on.

"Dad has a kind of cancer," Mom said. I wasn't sure what that meant but it didn't sound good.

"What's that?"

"It means that some of the cells in Dad's body are reproducing too fast and causing problems in his body."

I still didn't understand. Dad seemed pretty dazed and confused.

"The cancer is in his lymph nodes, which are growing too big and causing problems with his nerves, which is why he has been having back pains."

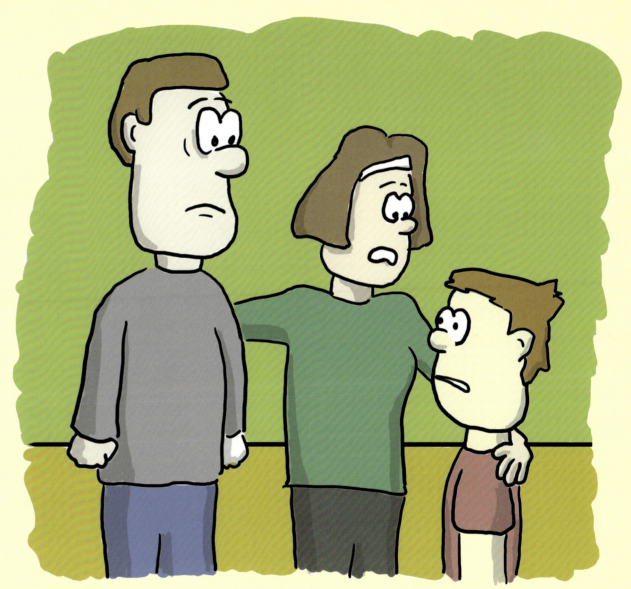

"I'm going to be all right," Dad said. I knew he was trying to sound brave, and he didn't want me to worry, but I could tell he was scared. "The chances for a cure are really good. Mario Lemieux had it, and he came back to play for the Pittsburgh Penguins."

Finally something I could understand. I'm a big hockey fan, and I knew that Mario was one of the best ever.

"The doctor says that the chemotherapy should get rid of the cancer."

Chemotherapy?!

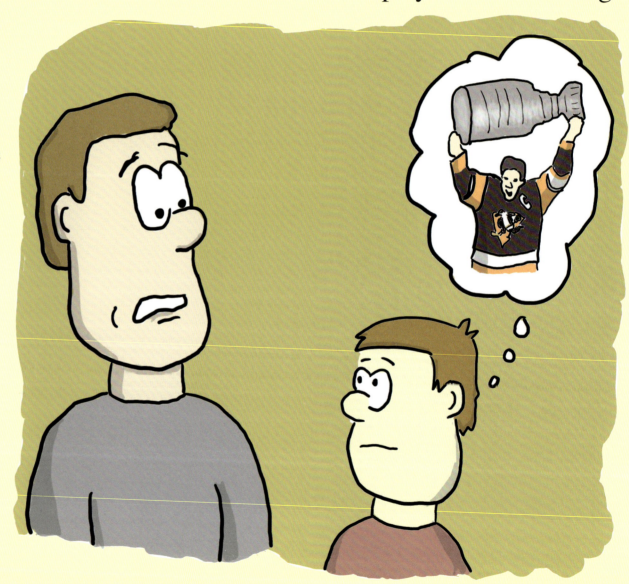

Mario Lemieux had a cancer called lymphoma. There are two types of lymphoma, Hodgkin's and Non-Hodgkin's, and they, like leukemia, are called "blood cancers," because they attack the blood, bone marrow or lymph system. Some other famous people who had lymphoma include:

Jacqueline Kennedy Onassis, former First Lady
Roger Maris, baseball great
Gene Autry, country western legend
Joey Ramone, Rock and Roll Hall of Famer
Charles Lindbergh, aviation legend
Paul Allen, Microsoft cofounder and owner of NBA Portland Trailblazers
Andrés Galarraga, All-Star baseball player
Jonathan Alter, Newsweek senior editor
Joe Ferguson, NFL quarterback
Larry Lucchino, CEO of the Boston Red Sox
Merril Hoge, NFL running back and ESPN analyst
Dave Roberts, Major League outfielder
Joe Vide, Major League Soccer star
Jon Lester, threw no-hitter for Boston Red Sox after being treated for lymphoma
Ethan Zohn, "Survivor: Africa" winner
Saku Koivu, long-serving captain of Montreal Canadians
Joe Andruzzi, NFL lineman
Mr. T, television personality
Michael C. Hall, television personality

Chemotherapy?!

Chemotherapy is the term for the chemicals used to stop cancer cells from growing. More than half of all people diagnosed with cancer receive chemotherapy, and it helps treat cancer in millions of patients.

Most times chemotherapy is given in doses over several months, often through a needle in a vein or by a pill that is swallowed, depending on which drug is used.

Although chemotherapy is good because it destroys cancer cells, it cannot tell the difference between a cancer cell and some healthy cells. That means chemotherapy kills all of a body's fast-growing cells, like hair and blood cells. That is why people on chemotherapy lose their hair and have a greater chance of getting sick without white blood cells to fight infections.

Mom took Dad to get chemotherapy the next week. I didn't get to go, and it didn't sound like fun. He had to sit in a chair for hours with a needle in his arm while nurses put the medicine in his body.

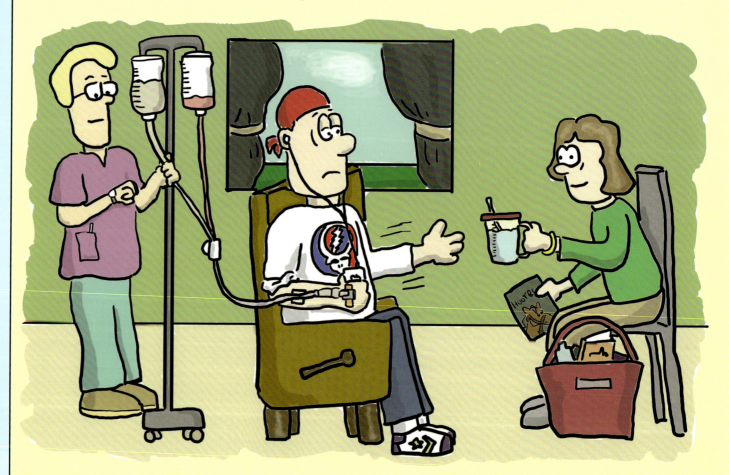

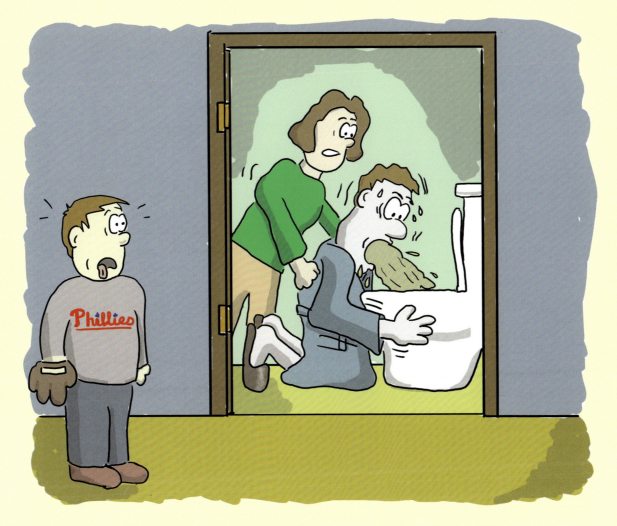

The medicine was really strong, and it made Dad feel worse than the cancer. When he came home he didn't look so good, and all he could do was lay on the couch. Things got worse that night. Dad started to throw up and couldn't stop hiccupping. I hate the hiccups. He threw up a bunch of times.

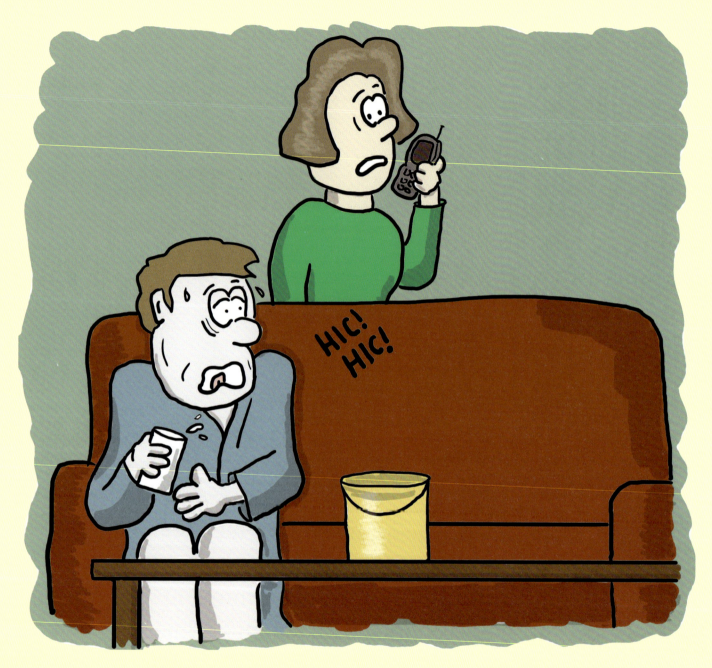

Mom was getting worried, and she decided to take him to the emergency room.

Our neighbor came over to stay with me until my grandparents could get here. We watched some baseball on TV, but I was having a hard time not thinking about Dad. When I went to bed, Mom and Dad were still at the hospital.

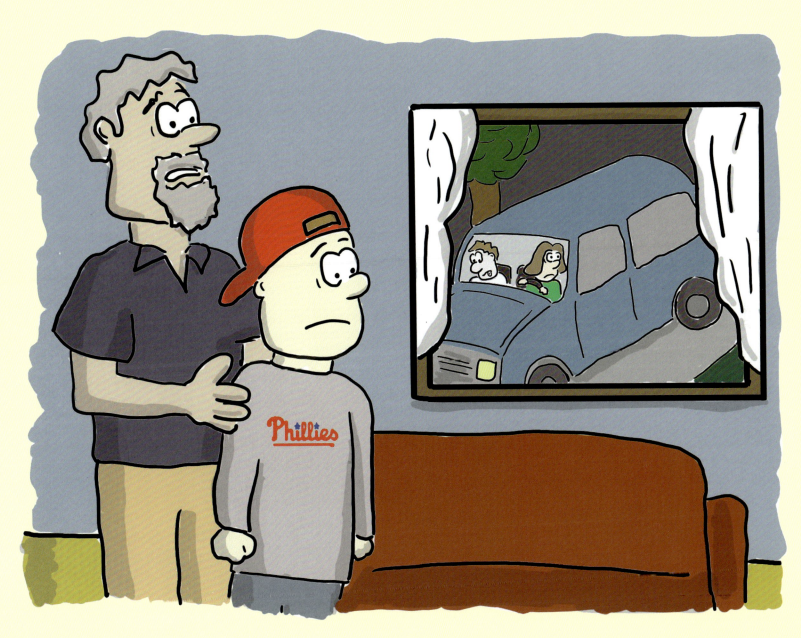

The next morning when my parents were still not back from the hospital, I was scared. My grandparents were going to take me to my soccer game that morning, but I didn't want to go. I wanted to cry. Grandpa told me that it was all right to be worried, but Dad was going to be all right, and he would want me to play my game.

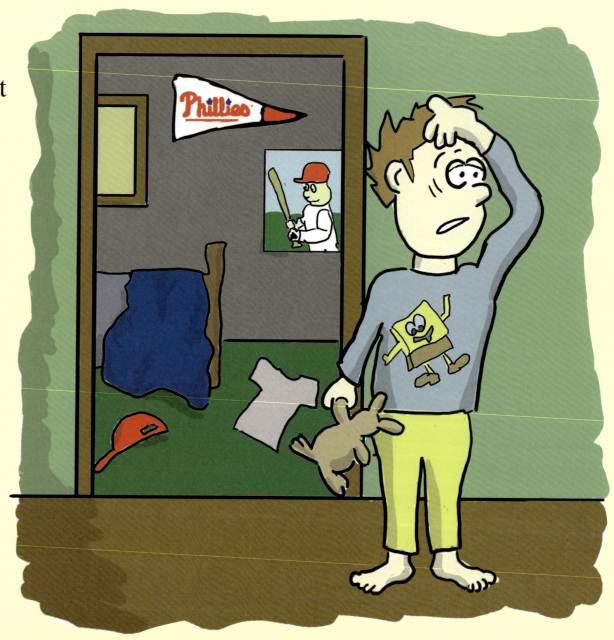

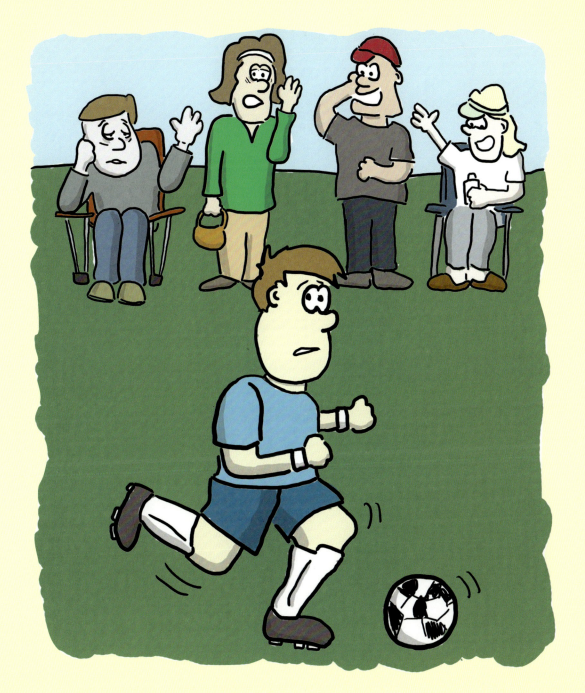

As the game started I was having a hard time getting into it. Then I saw Dad and Mom walking across the field. Dad looked sick and weak, but he had come straight from the hospital to watch my game.

I was so glad to see him. I tried to play my best.

After the game, Dad went home and watched football for the rest of the day. That wasn't so unusual for him, but he definitely wasn't the same. Usually he hoots and hollers whenever his team scores. Today he didn't seem to care.

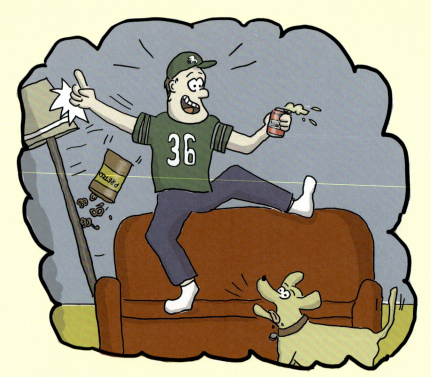

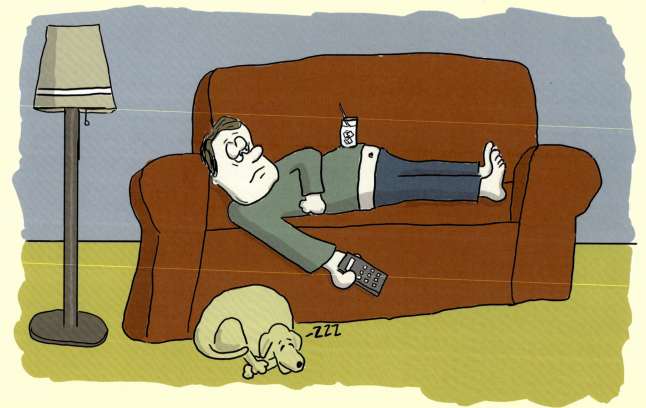

That's how things went for the next couple of months. Dad didn't leave the house a lot of days. After school he didn't have the energy to play street hockey with me. Some nights he even went to bed before me. Mom was getting tired, too. She had to do a lot more things around the house. We both had to do more chores since Dad wasn't able to help as much.

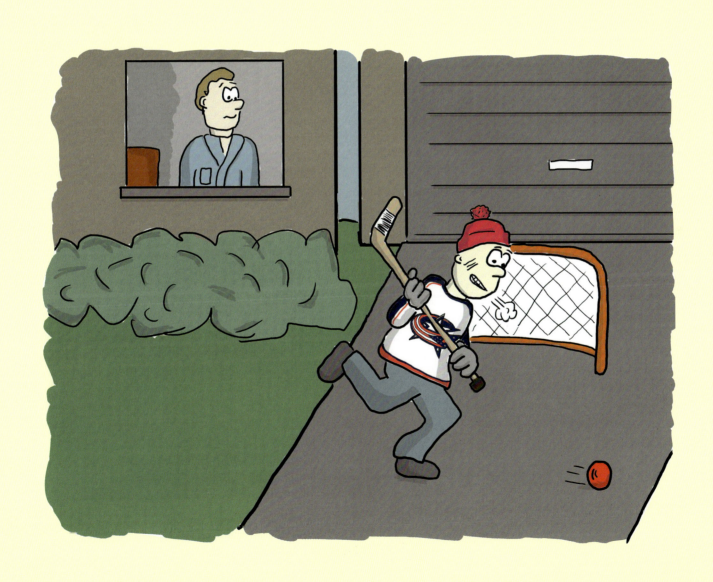

Dad had to go to chemotherapy every couple weeks, and pretty soon he started to look different. ***He started to lose his hair!***

Dad always said that I made his hair turn gray, but now it was falling out every time that he took a shower. It was on his pillow when he woke up in the morning.

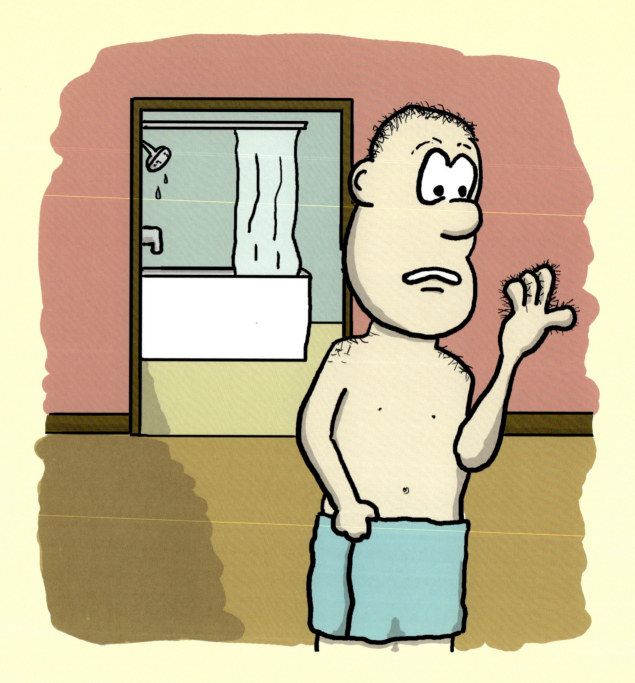

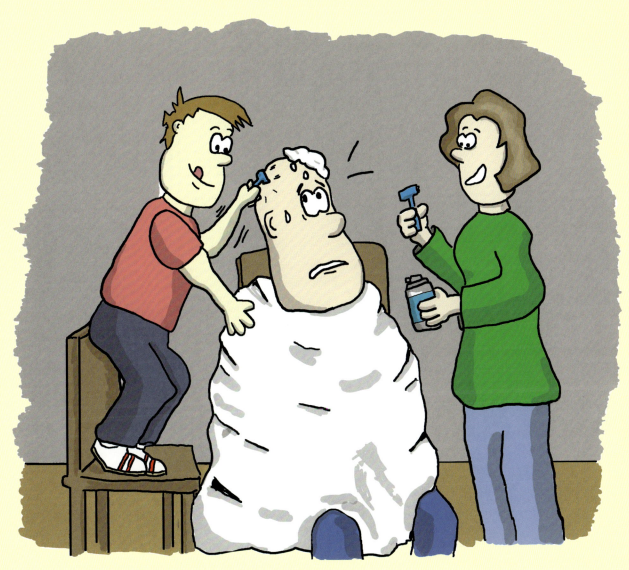

Finally, he said he'd had enough. Mom and I shaved his head. I had to be careful with the razor, but it was kind of fun. When we were done his head was a smooth as a bowling ball!

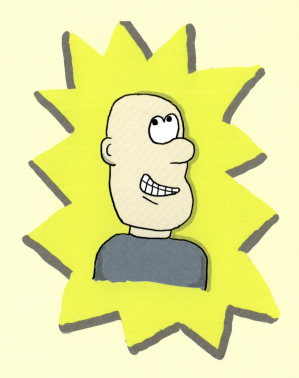

Dad said being bald was hard to get used to. He looked weird, and sometimes I had to look at him twice to make sure it was really him. I wanted to shave my head, too, but Dad said that it was cold to be completely bald, and as a hockey player I spent a lot of time in cold ice rinks.

So, I asked Mom to give me a crew cut. Dad and I got matching Phillies hats. We wore them everywhere we went.

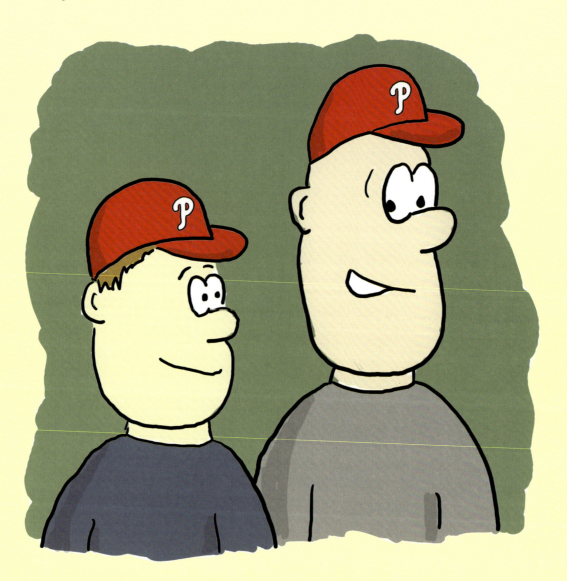

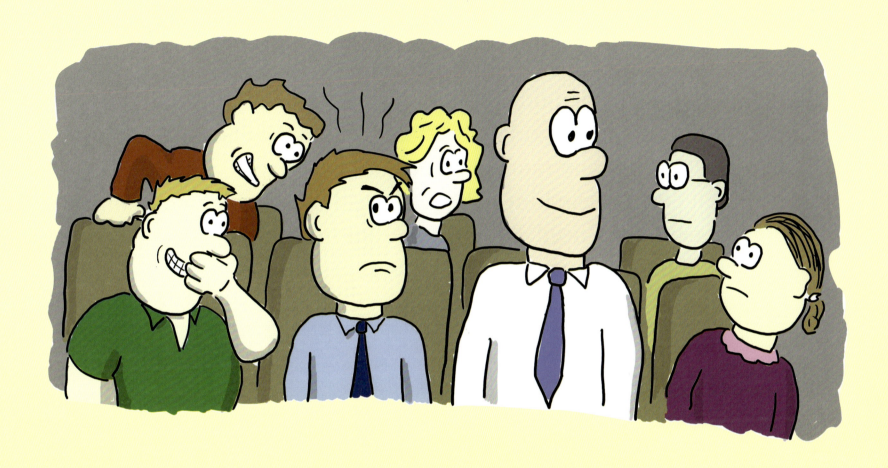

On the day of our class trip to a play, Dad was feeling pretty good, so he went with us to the fancy theater downtown.

It was the kind of thing you dress up for, so we had to leave our baseball hats at home. Most of my classmates hadn't seen my Dad in a while, and they pointed at him when he showed up at the theater without his hair. Some of the kids even laughed at him. It didn't seem to bother him—he was laughing with them.

While going through chemotherapy, it was important that Dad didn't get sick, because his body was working so hard to fight the cancer. That meant Dad couldn't volunteer any more at my school, since kids carry lots of germs, and that could make him sick pretty easily. I missed having him at school, but I knew that I needed to be brave for him.

At home we made sure to wash our hands a lot—*a whole lot*.

Chemotherapy and the Immune System

Chemotherapy kills cells that divide rapidly, like most cancer cells. Unfortunately, this also destroys some of the white-blood cells that make up our immune system, which defends our bodies against sickness and disease.

That means people undergoing chemotherapy should avoid sick people and wash their hands a lot to wash away germs. If a patient gets sick it takes longer to recover, and chemotherapy might have to be stopped to let the body to recover.

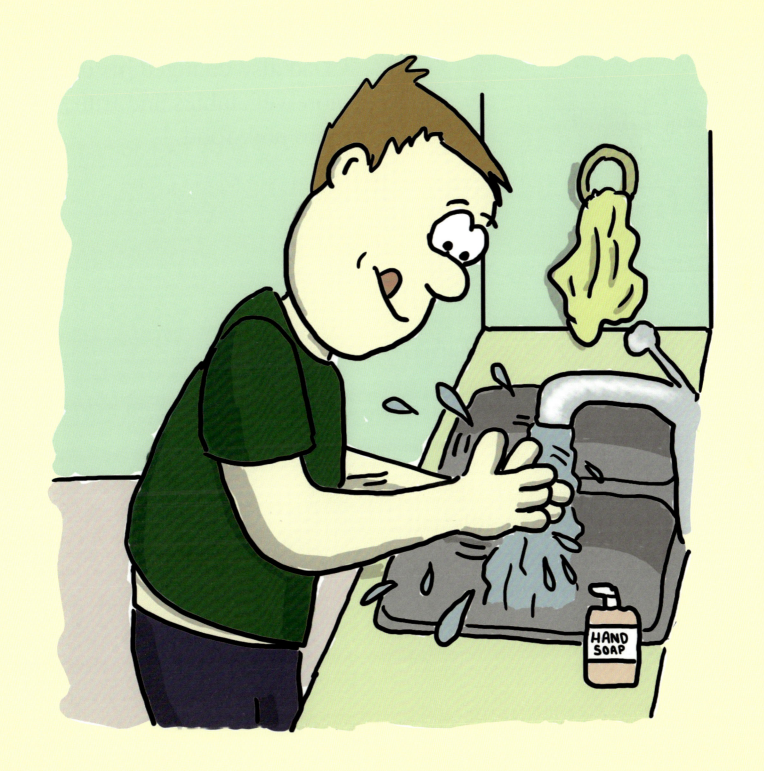

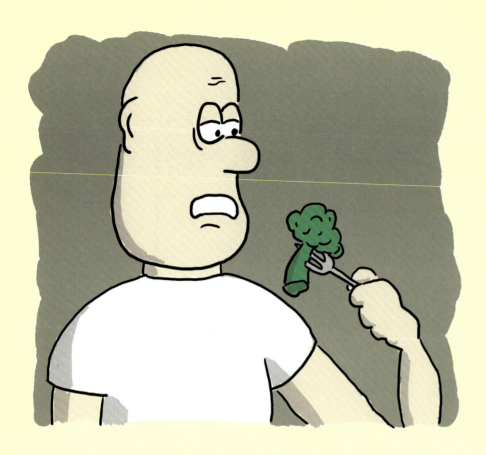

Dad also changed his diet to eat more vegetables and fruit, and no more junk food.

He also took lots of pills and medicine, which didn't look like it tasted very good.

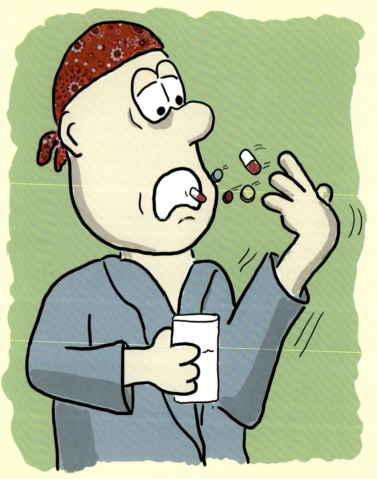

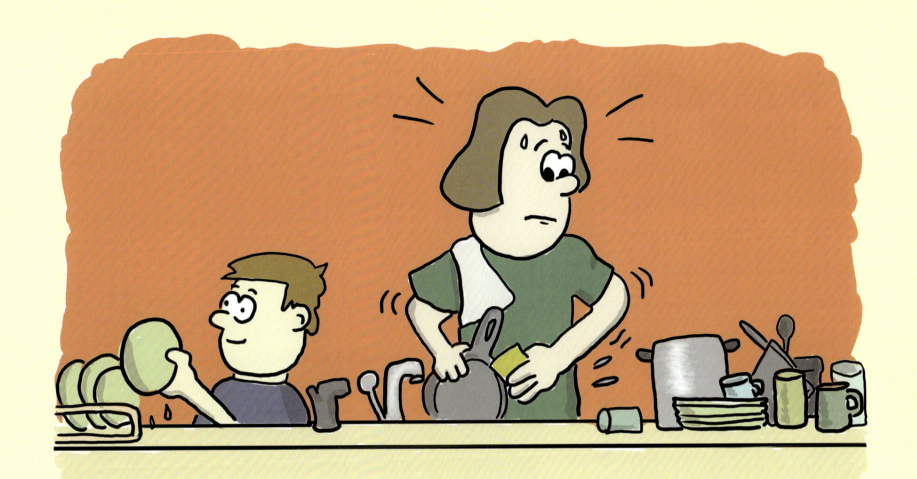

We didn't eat out in restaurants much, because we had to make sure that his food was clean and healthy.

Mom spent a lot of time cooking and cleaning.

This went on for months and months. His doctor said the chemotherapy was fighting the cancer—and winning—but Dad was getting more and more tired. Sometime I had to get rides to hockey practice with my friends. He tried to make it to all of my games, but sometimes he couldn't, and I tried to understand when he didn't have the strength.

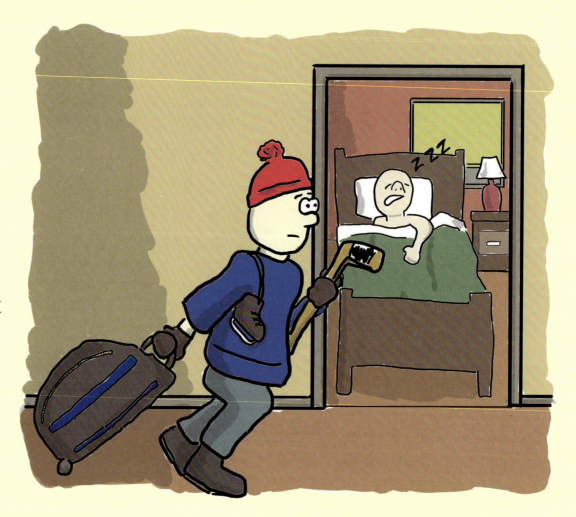

"Stay positive, and everything will work out," Dad kept saying, but I could tell he wasn't too happy.

He was never really sick before his cancer, and he didn't like hanging around the house. We didn't wrestle or play around like we used to, and he seemed pretty sad.

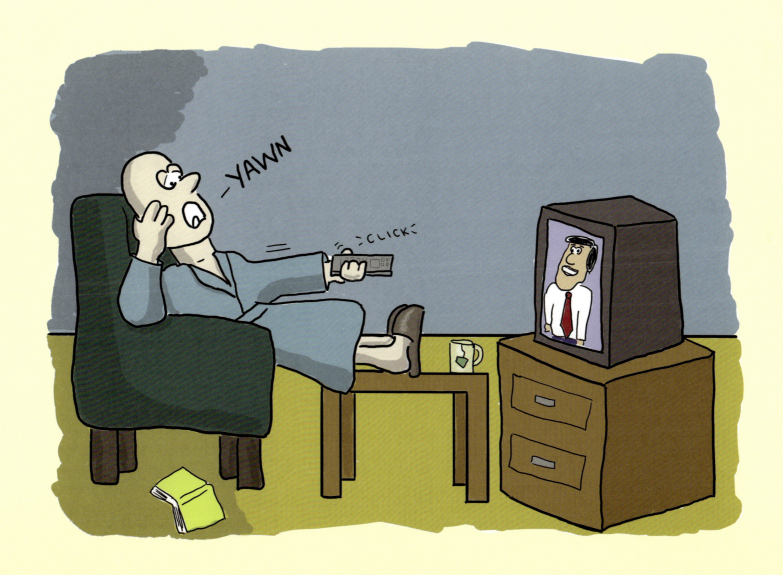

But then things started to turn around. The Phillies made the World Series–and they won the whole thing! I even got to stay up to watch the final game.

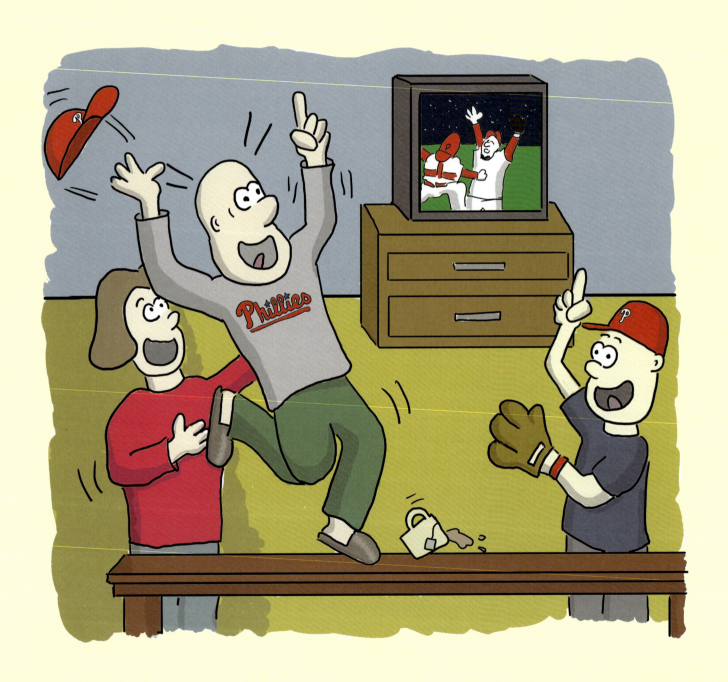

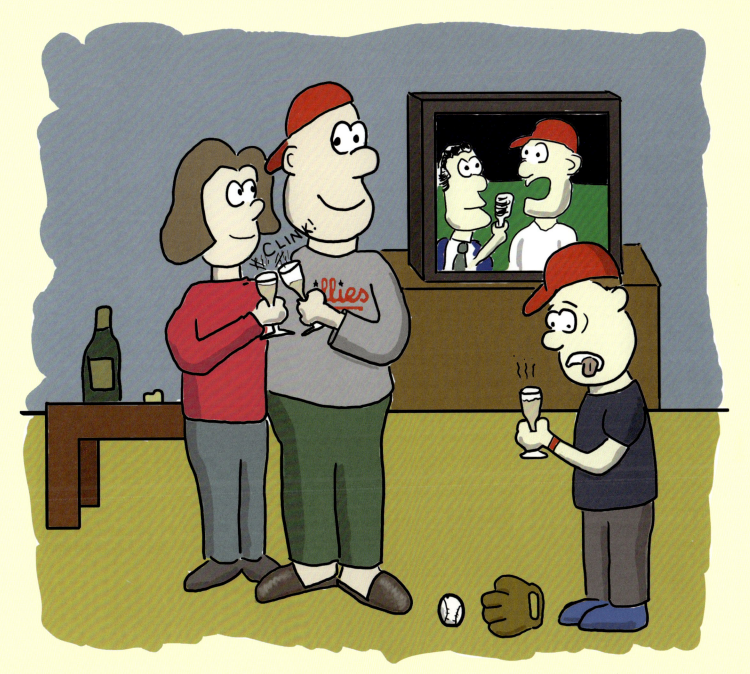

I hadn't seen him so happy in a long time.
Mom and Dad even let me taste champagne. *Yuck!*

Then Dad started to regain some strength. He played basketball with his friends and, although he got tired quickly, his doctor said the exercise was good for him.

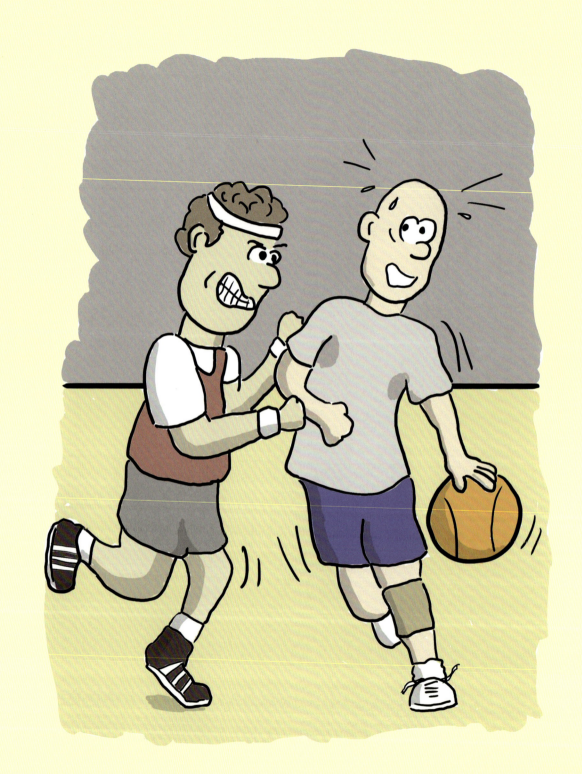

After six months, we finally got the news we wanted to hear. The cancer was gone. Everyday Dad seemed more like himself. He even started skating with me again.

I'd like to say things are back to normal, but I think this is our new normal. Every few months Dad goes for tests at the doctor to make sure the cancer hasn't come back. Mom still makes him eat healthy food and take vitamins—now she even makes me do it!

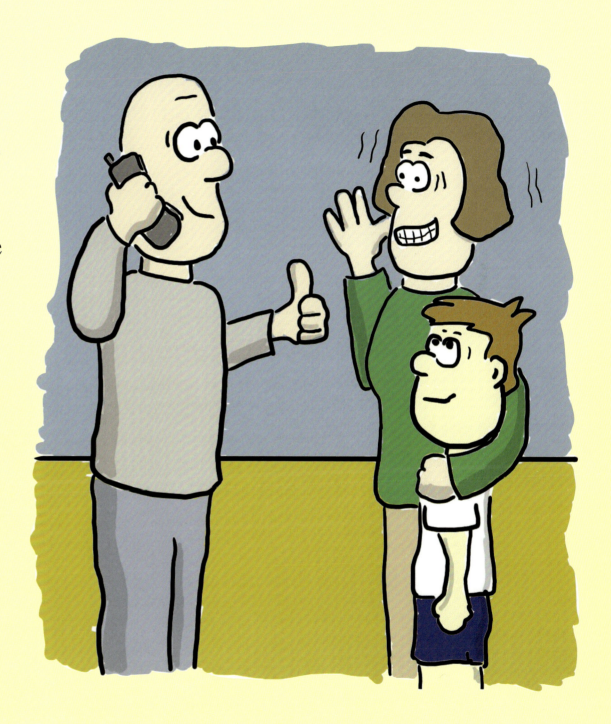

And just about every day when we go outside to play catch, we still put on our Phillies hats.

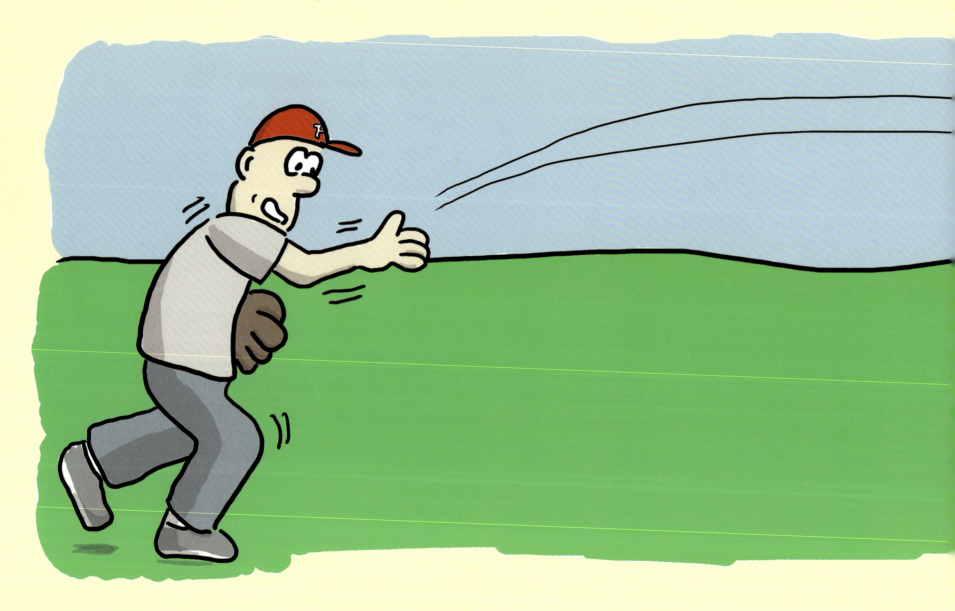

We hope they win the World Series again—*but this time when Dad has hair*.

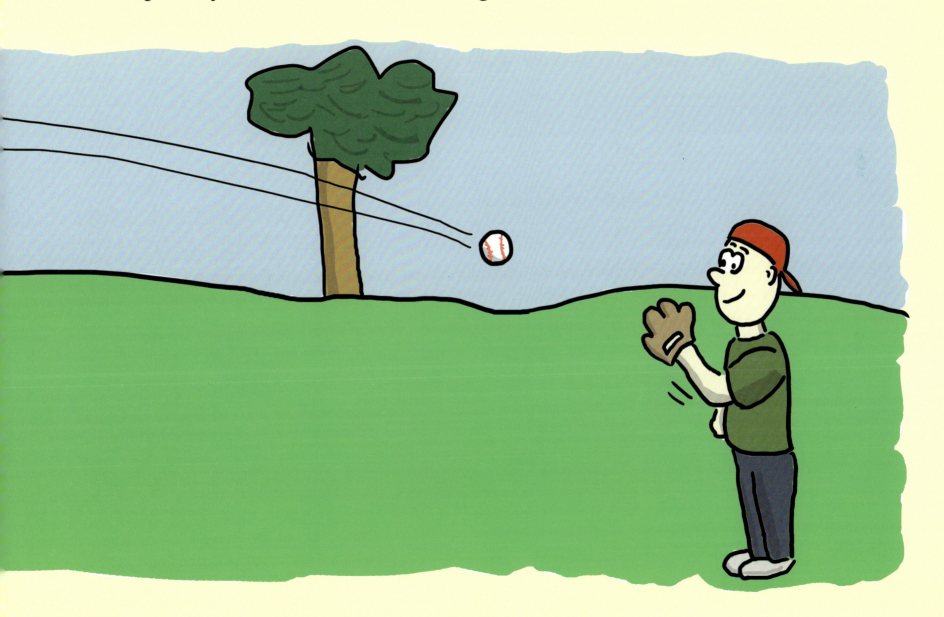

Resources

The Lymphoma & Leukemia Society
http://www.leukemia-lymphoma.org/
Dedicated to supporting people who face blood cancers.

Lymphoma Research Foundation
www.lymphoma.org
Dedicated to funding research to find a cure for lymphoma.

Patients Against Lymphoma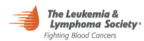
www.lymphomation.org
Provides a helping hand from patient to patient by sharing evidence-based information and voicing patient perspectives in the fight against lymphoma.

American Cancer Society
http://www.cancer.org
The United States' most well-known entity for cancer information.

LIVESTRONG
http://www.livestrong.org/
Started by cancer survivor and seven-time Tour de France winner Lance Armstrong to provide resources and support for cancer patients and their families.

Oncolink
http://www.oncolink.org/index.cfm
Founded by University of Pennsylvania cancer specialists with a mission to help cancer patients, families, health care professionals and the general public get free and accurate cancer-related information.

Hockey Fights Cancer
www.nhl.com
A joint initiative by the National Hockey League and the National Hockey League Players' Association to raise money and awareness for the fight against cancer.

Brian Kraft is a graphic artist and cartoonist based in Columbus Ohio. He was diagnosed with Non-Hodgkin's Lymphoma in September 2008 and has been cancer-free since January 2009.

This is his first book and hopefully his last one about having cancer. He currently enjoys a full head of hair.

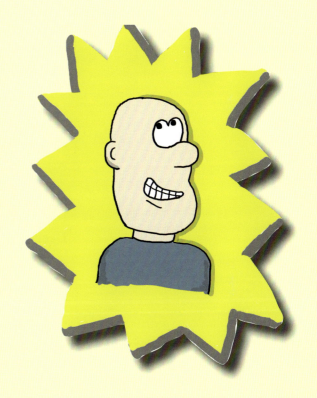

To Nicki and Danny. I wouldn't be here without you.
And to all our family and friends who never let us feel like we were alone.

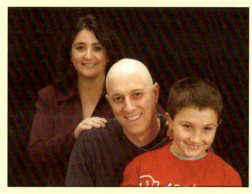

December 2008

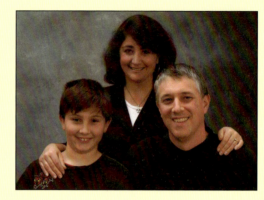

December 2009